Preface

Welcome to the journey of holistic healing and well-being. In this book, we delve into the profound connection between the body, mind, and soul, exploring how practices such as meditation, yoga, exercises, and nutrition can harmonize and revitalize these essential aspects of our being.

In today's fast-paced world, we often find ourselves caught in the whirlwind of stress, imbalance, and disconnection. Our bodies ache, our minds race, and our souls yearn for nourishment. Yet, amidst the chaos, there exists a path to restoration, a path illuminated by ancient wisdom and modern science alike.

Through the pages of this book, we embark on a transformative journey toward wholeness and vitality. We'll uncover the transformative power of meditation, guiding you through practices that quiet the mind, cultivate mindfulness, and unlock inner peace. We'll explore the ancient discipline of yoga, tapping into its ability to strengthen the body, increase flexibility, and foster spiritual growth.

But healing extends beyond the realms of the mind and body; it encompasses the nourishment of our very essence, our soul. Through introspection and self-discovery, we'll nurture our spiritual well-being, connecting with the deepest parts of ourselves and finding solace in the present moment.

Furthermore, we'll delve into the importance of physical activity, exploring exercises that invigorate the body, boost energy levels, and enhance overall health. Coupled with a well-balanced diet and proper nutrition, these practices form the cornerstone of holistic wellness, fueling our bodies with the nutrients they need to thrive.

As you embark on this journey, remember that healing is not a destination but a continuous process—a journey of self-discovery, growth, and transformation. May this book serve as a guide, illuminating your path toward radiant health, inner peace, and a harmonious union of body, mind, and soul.

With gratitude and blessings,

Dr Sheetal Chaudhary

About Author

Sheetal Chaudhary is a dedicated healer and advocate for holistic well-being. As a doctor by profession, she has spent years witnessing the intricate interplay between physical health, mental well-being, and spiritual vitality. Her passion for integrative medicine led her to explore the transformative power of practices such as meditation, yoga, and nutrition in restoring balance and vitality to the body, mind, and soul.

During the challenging times of the Covid-19 pandemic, Sheetal faced various obstacles, including navigating lockdowns and adapting to new modes of healthcare delivery. It was amidst these trials that she found solace and inspiration in the healing arts, ultimately leading her to pen this book.

Sheetal's journey toward healing is deeply personal. At the tender age of 8, she experienced the profound loss of her father, who battled blood cancer (leukaemia) with courage and grace. His resilience and unwavering spirit served as a beacon of inspiration, igniting Sheetal's passion for medicine and instilling in her a profound sense of purpose.

Sheetal holds her family dear to her heart, cherishing the memories of her beloved father and the unwavering support of her mother, Kamlesh Devi. She finds joy in the company of her brothers, Mohit Chaudhary and Mayank Chaudhary, and her sister, Ritu Chaudhary. Alongside her brother-in-law, Sushant Chaudhary, Sheetal shares a deep bond with her niece and nephew, Nirvi and Nirvaan.

In addition to her human family, Sheetal finds companionship and solace in the memories of her late dogs, Ellie and Bruno, who brought immeasurable joy and love into her life.

Through her writing, Sheetal seeks to share the wisdom she has gleaned from her experiences and inspire others to embark on their own journey toward healing and wholeness.

This book is dedicated to the memory of Sheetal's father, a loving husband, father, and friend, whose spirit continues to inspire and guide her every step of the way. He was a man of remarkable character, known for his kindness, generosity, and unwavering dedication to helping others. His influence has deeply shaped Sheetal's journey toward healing and serves as a constant source of inspiration in her life's work.

Connect with Sheetal Chaudhary:
She8just@gmail.com

Follow Sheetal on social media:
https://www.instagram.com/sheetal_chaudhary11_?igsh=MW5kc3A5OGVvcnY2MQ==

HEAL YOUR BODY MIND AND SOUL

DIMENSIONS OF HEALTH

1.Physical Dimension:- **a. All the organs of the body are of proportionate in size.**

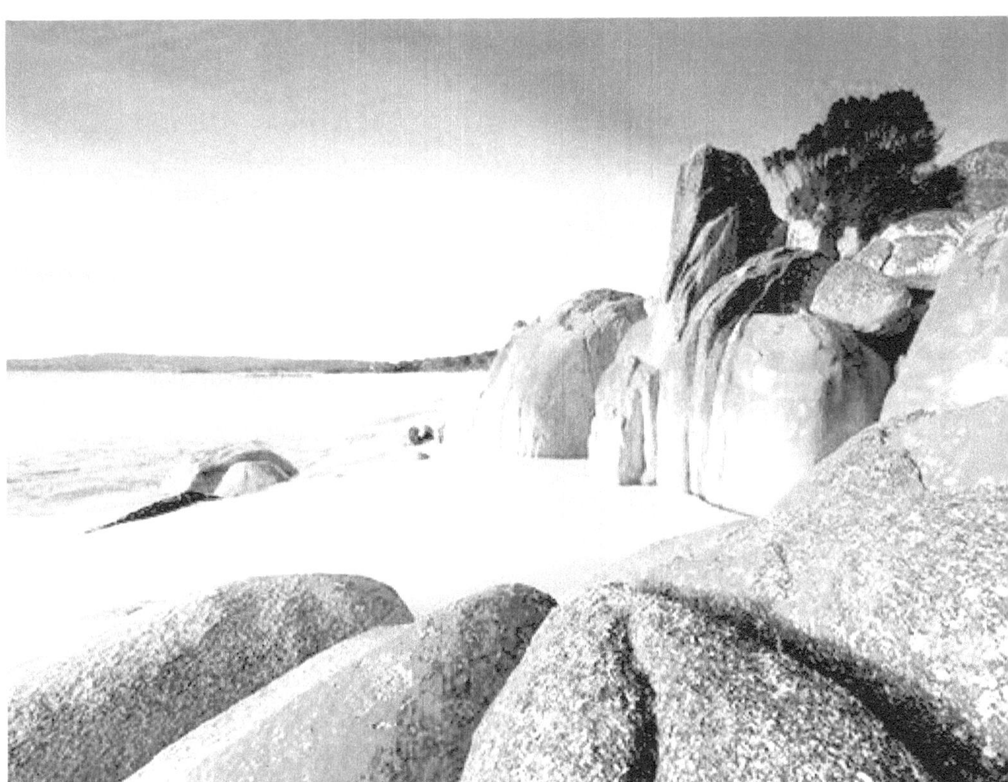

b. Body we'll clothed with firm flesh.

c. Good appetite, regular activity of bowels and bladder.

d. Coordinate bodily movements.

e. Sound sleep.

f. Pulse, B.P, R.R , exercise tolerance are normal and according to age and sex.

2.MENTAL DIMENSION

a. A state of balance Between the individual and the surrounding world, a state of harmony between oneself and the others, a coexistence between the realities of the self and that of the other people and that of the environment.

b. Free from internal conflicts, he is not at "war" with himself.

c. Well adjusted with others.

d. Searches for identity.

e. Has a strong sense of self esteem.

f. Faces problem and tries to solve them intelligently.

3.social dimension:- a. Harmony and integration within the individual between each individual and other members of society or environment in which they live.

b. It is the ability to see oneself as a member of large society.

4.spiritual dimension:-a. Having meaning and purpose in life b. commitment to some higher being. C. Having integrity, principles and ethics.

5.Other dimensions:-

a. Emotional

b. Vocational

c. Philosophy

d. Cultural

e. Educational

f. Nutritional

g. Curative etc.

These dimensions function and interact with each other.

Concept of well being:- well being of an individual or group of individuals have objective and subjective components. The objective components are generally known by the term "standard of living" or level of living ".The subjective component of well being is referred to as "Quality of life".

1.standard of living:-According to WHO-"Income and occupation, standards of housing, sanitation and nutrition, the level of provision koolof health, education, recreation, and other services may all be used individually as measures of socio-economic status and collectively as an index of the "standard of living".

2.level of living:-The parallel term for standard of living used in United Nations documents is "level of living".It consists of nine components. Health, food, consumption, education, occupation, working conditions, housing social Security, clothing, recreation and leisure and human right.

3.Quality of life:- quality of life was defined by WHO as "the condition of life resulting from the combination of the effect of the complete range of factors such as those determining health, happiness (including comfort in the physical environment and a satisfying occupation), education social and intellectual attainment s, freedom of action, justice and freedom of expression".

A recent definition of quality of life is as follows. "a composite measures of physical, mental and social well being as perceived by each individual or by group of individuals- That is to say happiness, satisfaction and

gratification as it is experienced in such life concerns as
health, marriage, family work, financial situation,
educational opportunities, self-esteem, creativity
belongingness and trust in others".

DAILY ROUTINE

Everyday whatever we eat done for our well being is known
as DALY ROUTINE.

Wake up early in the morning and follow all the rules which
makes you healthy comes under the Daily routine.

Importance of Daily Routine:- It is a first aim of Ayurveda.
"protect the health of healthy person" and Daily Routine
also have the same aim to protect the body, soul and mind
of the healthy person.

1.Wake up early in the morning:-In Ayurveda it is called
Brhammurata, "Brham" means Knowledge. For worship
God it is the best time.

2.Always went to the Loo according to your body. Night
food should be digested .

Uses of exercise:- Body feels lightness, increase the
working capacity of the body , Body feels strengthen,
walking, jogging, swimming, Gymnastics, sports and games
etc are Health increasing ideas.

1.Body's muscles became strong and flexible. This help in
daily routine activities.

2.Blood flows normally in body.

3.Body's different organs like Respiratory organs, Heart (cardiovascular system) Digestive system, Nervous system, etc, will work in better manner.

4.Mental Depression will never happen.

5.Inspite of all these diseases some diseases like obesity, HTN, Diabetes, Hypothyroidism etc. can be cured.

Daily taking Bath can make people energetic, people live long life. It reduces lethargy, excessive sweating, foul smell from body. It energies the whole body and power of body increases.

According to Ayurveda Acharya Shushrut who is also Known as the father of surgery he introduces the Surgery to the whole world. He belongs to India. Shushrut said that bathing strengthens the heart and it gave more power and energies the senses. It reduces fatigue from the body and purified the blood and increases the appetite of the body.

Peoples who are suffering from the following diseases should not take bath:-a.Diarrhoea b. Fever. C. Ear disease D. Eye disease E. Indigestion F. After taking meal.

Most of the people are washing their hairs from hot water which is very harmful for the eyes and for hairs only the cold water is good for body. Peoples of India mostly taking Bath from cold water even in winter also. In Ayurveda Acharya's said cold water is recommended for people in spite of hot water . It is also said by shushrut (father of surgery) in Ayurveda that we should take bath according to the season. Taking bath from cold water is good for lower part of the body. It gives strengthen to the whole pelvic Region of the body.

Washing of legs reduces fatigue and even disease also It clean the eyes and make it more powerful. In Ayurveda there is a big role of applying paste of medicated herbs which is known as "lape"in Sanskrit.This "lape" or paste of medicated herbs is applied on the whole body after taking Bath. It has a pleasant fragrance which removes the sweating, foul smell from the body and it increases the power of the body. But it is applied only according to the season. In Ayurveda there is also a very important role of wearing clothes. It is said by Achaaryas like "charak" who is also known as the first physician of india. He wrote about so many diseases and their symptoms and their methods of cure. By wearing clean clothes person energies their whole body. It increases their life and reputation according to Acharya charak. In India the money is compared with the goddess "laxmi.So In Diwali festival most of the people in India worship the goddess laxmi. So people of India wearing new clothes on the occasion of Diwali and celebrate it by giving sweets and gifts to their near and dear. So it is symbolises with the Laxmi also by wearing clean clothes. Wearing fragranted materials like jewelry called "Mala" in Hindi increases the life of the people it gave power to people, wearing jewelry indicates in India that the person is rich and it symbolises the long life of person. It makes heart happy.

In evening it is very important to do the Yoga everyday. According to the Acharya Bhavan Mishra in evening taking food, reading book, sleeping, walking on road. These things should not be done. Eating food in evening Can lead to the food disease, doing study in evening can lead to the decrease in wealth and can decrease the life span of the person.

Taking food in evening:-In evening person should take less food because it takes long time to digest at night. One should take very lite food which is easily digested. After eating less and healthy food one should remember the God and should went to the bed.

How to sleep:-The place of sleep should be clean and should not be congested.

According to Ayurvedic principles people is equal to the whole world. All the feelings which is present in the whole world is also present in one person's body. It means when the season is changed the changes in the body of the person will be happened. Peoples should take food according to the seasons. Peoples who take food according to the season will always be the healthy person and will never be suffered by any kind of disease.

How to behave:- peoples who want betterment for their body and soul should follow the truth path called "sadvrita In Sanskrit. Peoples who follow sadvrita had benefits:-
1.Arogyata(free from disease)

2. Indriyavijya(victory on senses).

Inspite of all these that person live for 100 years. That person became healthy and wealthy . He developed brotherhood among all the peoples. By doing good karmas he went to the heaven.

Importance:-Diseases has 3 causes 1.Do not have control on senses (Asatmayindriyarth San yoga). It means all the peoples have senses like smell, touch, by watching through eyes, hearing, taste. So when anything happened wrong with one of the senses so the disease will appeared in human body.

Socially development:- To grow socially follow these things in your life :- 1.Always speak truth at a right time and speak nicely meaningful and accurate talks to other peoples. Always care about our old peoples, teachers.

Not to Do:- Never said bad words to old peoples, to their parents and teachers. Never feel jealousy by watching others success . Never went to walk at late night. Never make friendship with stupid and greedy peoples. Never see fault in others. Never do beaching of others

Mental development:- For the betterment of good mental status one should follow these points:-

1.Always make distance from jealousy and fighting

2.Always tries to calm down to angry peoples

3.Always feel happy from heart

4.If anyone says wrong to you never said wrong word to them back.

5.Be kind to everyone whether it is an animal or a human being or a bird.

Not to do:-1.Never speak lie

2.Never make enemies

3.Never lose trust to your family members

4.Never be impatient

5.Never do wrong things

6.Never trust people easily

7.Never think so much to whole day

8.Never feel jealousy, never feel angry, never be proudy, and greedy

Cleanness:- In the morning and evening daily take bath. Always clean your legs and hands

Always wear clean clothes. Always comb your hairs regularly. Do regularly oiling of your feet, Nose, head, Ear.

Not to do:-Always cover your face during Yoneing, sneezing.

Exercise related good habits:-Never do climbing of mountain hills regularly.

Never climb the trees. Never sit on your foot for long time.

Never move your body parts in wrong manner.

Food Related Good Habits:--Never eat food before bathing, before worship the God,

Before washing the hand and face, Never eat food with dirty hands, never eat

Food in dirty utensils. According to Ayurveda never eat curd at night.

Never eat high quantity of food at night because it takes long time to digest

As we all know now a days Intermediate fasting is in trend for the people's who

Want to loose their weight should follow the timing of eating the food.

Study Related Good Habits:- If there is any occasion and festival

It is contraindicated for study according to Ayurveda. In

Evening or late night study is not allowed according to Ayurvedic Acharyas because

It gives pressure on the eyes to read or write words. One should study frequently never

Skip the words, without pressure, without words, without teachers, never

Study with very loud or very slow voice.

Work Related Good Habits:- Never disobey the working hours

Never work at strange site.

Never be the person who work late night.

Never be so happy when you get success or never be so sad when you are unsuccessful

In your work.

Always start work for good reason. Never sit by knowing you have done enough.

Mental health is a balanced development of the individual's personality and emotional attitudes which enable him to live harmoniously with his follow men. A mentally healthy person has 3 main characteristics

1.He feels comfortable about himself and feels secure. He

Neither under-estimate nor over estimate his own ability

2.He feels right towards others and love to others. He

Is able to like and trust others. He takes responsibility for

His neighbors and his fellows

3.He is able to meet the demand of life, solves the problems and

Take his own decisions. He sets reasonable goals for himself.

He is not bowled over by his own emotions of fear, anger, love,

Guilt etc.

Types of mental illness:-1.Major illness

2.Minor illness:-Neurosis(psycho-neurosis) :-
1.schizophernia(split personality)

2.manic depressive psychosis

3.paranoia

Prevention of Mental Illness:-1. Primary:-This consists of improving the social environment by better living conditions of the people.

2.secondary:-This consists of early diagnosis of mental illness

Through screening programmes in schools, industries, societies etc.

3.Tertiary:-To reduce the duration of mental illness and these

Reduces the stress for family and community

4.National mental health program:-It was launched in

7th plan 11 institutions have been identified for imparting training

In basic knowledge and skills in the field of mental health to the primary

Health care physicians .

Three pillars of health:- According to Ayurveda Body is made up of 3 pillars

1.vata

2.pitta

3.kaph

With these there are other pillars which helps to build the body.

Due to their use or misuse disease occurs

Food is one of the important pillar of health

The material which passes through the food pipe and digested

And gave nutrition to the different parts of body and escape them from any damage

Increase the capacity of the body and gives life is called food.

Importance of food:--As the whole world is made up of 5

Types of material like water, soil, air, and fire and sky same

As the food is also made up of 5 matcrials called

"Panchmahabhut" in Sanskrit language in Ayurveda.

Vedas and manuscripts have mentioned food as the "Brahms ".

In Vedas food gets very important. The very famous teacher or Acharya

Food borne disease:- A disease usually either infectious or toxic in nature, caused by agents that enter the body through the ingestion of food.

1.food borne intoxication:-a.Due to naturally occurring toxins in some foods

b. Lathyrism:-caused by intake of khessaridal (Lathyrism sativus) which have a neurotoxin viz., Beta oxalate amino alanine consumption of this pulse for long period of time (2-6) months causes neurodegenerative disorder characterized by progressive, permanent, spastic paraplegia (upper motor

neuron type of paralysis of both lower limbs), resulting in crippling deformity. This condition is called "Neuro lathyrism".

b. Epidemic dropsy:-Due to contamination of mustard or other oils

With argemone oil (seeds of Argemone maxicana-prickly poppy). Argemone has toxic alkaloid viz., sanguinarine which interferes with the oxidation of pyruvic acid. The symptoms are sudden non-inflammatory bilateral swelling of legs, associated with diarrhoea. Dyspepsia, cardiac failure and death may follow.

1.Due to toxins produced by certain fungi :-

a. Aflatoxin

b. Ergot

C. Fusarium

d. Due to toxins produced by some bacterias :-1.Botulism

2.staphylococus poisions

3.food borne chemical poisoning:-1.heavy metals e. g. Mercury (usually in fish), cadmium (in certain shelfish) and lead(in canned food)

4.oils, petroleum derivatives and solvents

5.Migrant chemicals from package materials

6.Asbestos

7.pestecide residues (DDT, BHC)

Food borne infections;-1.bacterial diseases-typhoid, food poisoning, cholera,

Streptococcus, staphylococus infection etc.

2.Viral diseases:-Hepatitis, gastroenteritis etc

3.parasites:-Ascariasis, Amoebiasis, taeniasis etc.

Classification of food:-1.classification by origin:-a.foods of animal origin

b. Foods of vegetable origin

C. Classification by chemical composition

D. Proteins

E. Fats

F. Carbohydrates

G. Vitamins

H. Minerals

Classification by predominant functions:-1.Body building foods e.g.milk,

Meat, poultry, fish, eggs, pulses, groundnuts etc.

2.Energy giving foods e.g.cereals, roots and tubers, fats and oils

3.protective foods:-vegetables, fruits, milk etc

Classification by nutritive value:-1.cereals and millets

2.pulses(legumes)

3.vegetables

4.Nuts and oil seeds

5.fruits

6.Animal foods

7.fats and oils

8.sugar and jaggery

9.condiments and spices

10.Miscellaneous foods

Classification by requirements:-a.Macro nutrients(proximate principles of food) –

Proteins, fats, carbohydrates

b. Micro nutrients(protective principles of food) -vitamins and minerals.

IDEAL FOOD:-Ideal food is also known as balanced diet.

Balanced diet is one which contains a variety of foods in such quantities

and proportions that the need of energy, amino acid, vitamins, minerals, fats,

Carbohydrates and other nutrients are adequatly met for maintaining health vitality and

General well being and also makes a small provision for extra nutrients to with stand short

Period of starvation.

Principles of balanced diet:-1.The daily requirement of protein should be met(15-20%) of total daily energy intake

2.Fat requirement should be limited to 20-30% of total daily energy intake, out of them saturated fat should be less than 10%.

3.Carbohydrates rich in naturals fibre should constitute the remaining of food energy.

4. The requirements of micro nutrients should be met.

5. Salt intake should be reduced to 5gms/day.

6. Junk foods such as colas, ketchup etc. Should be reduced.

The dietary pattern depending upon the climatic conditions of the region, economic capacity,

Religion, customs, tastes and habits of the people.

The requirements of different diet constituents is according to:-

1. Age

2. Sex

3. specific period e. g. Pregnancy and lactation

4. physical activity i.e., sedentary, moderate and heavy workers

5. According to diseases.

Social Aspects of Nutrition:-There are many social factors which influence the

State of nutrition in a society.

1. conditioning Influences:-In poor environmental conditions small children

May suffer from infections like diarrhoea, intestinal worms, measles, malaria, tuberculosis etc.

This infection causes malnutrition and malnutrition increases the chance of infections,

So a vicious cycle is established.

2.Cultural influences:-1.Certain food are not used by particular society due to their food

habits, customs, believes, traditions and attitudes .

2.personal likes and dislikes play an important role in the selection of food.

3.cooking method effects the nutritive value of food e. g., prolonged boiling in

Open pans and draining away the rice water at the end of cooking decreases the

Nutritive values.

3.Socio economic factors:-poverty, illiteracy, lack of knowledge about nutrition, lack

Of sanitation, large families etc. Cause malnutrition.

4.Food production:-Increased food production is responsible for increased food consumption

26

at family level but uneven distribution of food in country causes malnutrition inspite

Of good production of food.

5.Health and other services:-Nutritional surveillance, nutritional rehabilitation,

Nutritional supplementation and health education improve the level of nutrition in community.

Diseases due to malnutrition:- Malnutrition is a pathological state resulting from a relative or absolute deficiency or excess of one or more essential nutrients. It has 4 spectrum:-

1.Undernutrition:-Results when insufficient food is eaten over an extend period of time e. g. Low birth weight, PEM etc.

2.Imbalance:-Results when nutrients are not used in proper proportion.

3.Over nutrition:-Results when excessive food is eaten over an extend period of time

e. g. Obesity, diabetes mellitus.

4.specific deficiency:-Results from relative or absolute deficiency of a nutrients

e. g. Beri beri, rickets, anemia, scurvy, night blindness etc.

Vegetarian and Non vegetarian food:-

Vegetarian food:- Advantages:-

1.Easily available and cheaper

2.Easy to digest

3.Dietary fibers are provided only by vegetarian diet which are beneficial

In obesity, diabetes, coronary heart disease, hypertension, constipation,

Gall stone etc.

4.Vit C is mainly obtained from vegetarian diet

5.oils of vegetables are rich in polyunsaturated fatty acids which

Increases HDL and protest from cholesterol deposion (coronary heart disease)

Disadvantages:-1.Vegetables proteins are inferior to animal proteins

Because they are "biologically incomplete"(do not have all essential amino acids)

2.Bioavailability of plant source vitA, calcium and iron is less.

3.VitD, and B12 is not present is vegetarian diet.

4.To complete the diaper requirement vegetarians food should be

Taken in large amount.

NON Vegetarian diet:-1.Animal proteins are biologically complete

2.Inhibitors like oxalic acid, dietary fibres etc are not found so

Absorption of iron and calcium is good.

3.Vit A is found in recently form which has more bioavailability to B-carotene

In plants.

4.Vit D, B12 are found only in animal origin of food.

Disadvantages:-1.Non-vegeterian food is expensive and heavy

For digestion.

2.Animal fats are rich in saturated fatty acids, which increases

LDL and VIDEO, thus increases cholesterol and risk factor for

Atherosclerosis. So it is harmful in hypertension, CHD, diabetes, obesity etc.

3.Vit C is not present which leads to scurvy disease.

Food Hygiene:-Food is a potential source of infection and is

Liable to contaminated by micro-organisms. Food hygiene implies

In production handling, distribution and serving all types of food.

The primary aim of food hygiene is to prevent food poisoning and

Other food-borne illness. It includes milk, meat fish, egg, fruits, vegetable hygiene.

Meat hygiene:-1.tapeworm infections-by tinea soleuim, T.saginata, fasciola hepatica.

2.Bacterial infections:-Anthrax, tuberculosis, and food poisoning.

These diseases are produced due to use of infected, unboiled or semi boiled meat

The characters of good meat are:-

1.Neither pale pink nor a deep purple tinted

2.firm and elastic to touch not flaccid

3.Not slimy and of disagreeable odour

4.Reaction should be acidic not basic

5.Fat should be shiny.

Animals intended for slaughter are subjected to proper

Inspection by veterinary staff.

1.Antimortem inspection:-Emaciation, exhaustion, pregnancy

Sheep pox, foot rot, diarrhoea, febrile conditions, brucellosis,

Actinomycosis or other diseases

2.Postmortem inspection:- Cysticercus Boris, liver flukes,

Abscesses, hydatidosis, speticimia, tuberculosis, parasitic and
modular infection

Of liver and lungs.

Fruits and vegetables Hygiene :- 1.The fruits and vegetables which are consumed

Raw should be washed before eating

2.Handling should be hygienic.

3.Rotten fruits and vegetables should be discarded

4.cooked vegetables are free of pathogenic organisms .

SANITATION OF EATING PLACES :-1.They should be away

From open drain, stable, manure pit, excreta or other nuisance

2.Floor should be impervious to keep them clean

3.Walls upto 3feet should be smooth, corners to be rounded and impervious

4. At least 100 feet square area /10 person should be there

5.proper lighting and ventilation should be maintain

6.kitchen should be impervious, smooth and minimum 60 feet

Square of area.

7.A separate room with temperature control for storage

Use of condiments and spices in food and their effects on body:-

1.They include Asafoetida, cardamom, chillies, garlic, cloves, ginger, mustard, pepper, tamarind, turmeric etc

2.They are used to enhance the palatability of food and stimulate appetite.

3.The essential oils present in them have carminative properties and may aid in

Digestion.

4. Some of them are rich in particular nutrients e. g. Chillies are rich in turmeric and

Coriander are rich in iron.

5. Some of them have specific activity e. g. Garlic is hypolipidemic, turmaric is antiseptic and

Analgesic, cloves, ginger and pepper are useful in cough and cold

6. Excessive consumption of condemints may cause peptic ulcer.

YoGA:-etymology of yoga:-Yoga word is derived from the word Yujre yogae it means to connect, be one, or to unite etc. So, thus yoga means a person should know that he is a part of God.

Development of yoga:-The Basic knowledge of yoga is started from an ancient time.

Definition of yoga:-According to an ancient Upanishads "when 5 senses with mind and Mann became stable. Then this state is called yoga. In this state the person became desire less. This yoga exercise should be done again and again otherwise this state will be destroyed soon and will get again by doing yoga. Nobody can reach God from voice, view but by accepting the presence of God.

Bhagwat Geeta :-1. Be the same in success or unsuccessful in any work is called yoga.

33

Yoga :-1.Bahiranga yoga:-a.social ethics

b. Personal ethics

C. Postural practices

d. Respiratory practices

2.sensorial practice

3.Aantarang yoga:-a.concentration

b. Meditation

C. Realisation

Description of yoga in Ayurveda:- Soul when connected to senses and when

Senses connect to their work then happiness and sadness occurred.

1.Vajraasan:-This is an meditated Aaron. It is done after having food. It cures the digestive

Diseases

2.Ushtarasan:-This Aasan helps in digestion, constipation, backache, spondylitis etc.

34

3.Gomukhasan:-It makes legs muscles strongs and also helpful in diabetes

4.Sarvangh Asan:--It helps in thyroid gland related diseases. It maintain flow of blood circulation in head so that it reduces depression, increase memory power, excessive sleep, laziness

5.Bhujang Asan:-It increases the digestion. It destroyed all the diseases. It is very useful in liver and kidney disease and in sciatica also.

6.Dhanur Asan:-It reduces abdominal fat, It is helpful in kidney, diabetes

7.Padmasan:-It is the main meditated Aasan. It cures all types of diseases of the body.

8.Aardhchakra Asan:-It is useful in backache, sciatica and it makes muscles of back more strong.

9.Makar Asan:-It is useful in sciatica, backache, slip disc etc.

10.pawan mukt Asan:-The muscles of stomach became stronger, fat deposited on the belly reduces repedily the gas deposited on the belly got exist. It is helpful in obesity, diabetes, hyper, constipation etc.

Naturopathy:- It is a science of health believes in the natural way of healing.

It means body has the capacity to heal itself. This self healing mechanism is promoted by they use of natural

measures I. e, food, water, mud, air, Sundays, fasting, massage, relaxation etc.,

Mahatma Gandhi was the person who initiated and promoted the naturopathy in India.

The main object of naturopathy is to attain the positive health and cure the diseases by means of natural principles, by using air, Sundays, water, earth, food, fasting, massage etc.

Principles of Naturopathy:-1.Naturopathy is based on the healing power of nature. In which 5 basic elements I. e., space (Aakash, air, fire, water and earth and food are used for therapy.

In Naturopathy food is considered as medicine. In terms of Hippocrates "let food be thy medicine and medicine be thy food".

In Naturopathy patient is treated not the disease. It treats the body as whole on all

Aspects of health I. E, physical, mental, social, spiritual.

Cause of diseases are lowered vitality, abnormal components of blood and lymph. Germs

Are secondary cause of diseases.

Acute disease are our friends not the enemies, they are result of cleansing mechanism of the body. Chronic diseases are the outcome of wrong treatment and suppression of the acute disease.

Body heals itself by cleansing mechanism, a Naturopath only helps in this mechanism with the aid of natural things.

Food doesn't enhance the vitality, but build the body. Fasting helps the body to heal itself.

5 Basic elements in Naturopathy:-

The procedure of Naturopathy are based on the 5 basic elements:-

1.Earth

2.water

3.fire.

4.space.

5.Air

Importance of Naturopathy in present era:-

Prime importance of Naturopathy is that it uses the nature

As a healer so the therapy is cost less or cheap and there

Is no side effect as seen in the use of modern drugs. In the

Modern therapy the disease is suppressed, later it becomes chronic, but

Nature cure the patient gets power to detoxify the morbid matter

Collected in the body which causes the disease.

1.what is considered Natural in Naturopathy and Ayurveda:-

Naturopathy utilizes the ingredients of nature-earth or

Mud, water, sunlight or other forms of heat, fasting, fruits

And vegetables. These substances are used because they are

Found in nature. Naturopathy considered these as Natural

For our body, healing. Holistic Ayurvedic medicine considered

the balance of 3 humors (catalog, pitta, kapha) , seven tissues

And sub tissues, the metabolic and excretory substances as

Other good qualities with innate universal appeal are considered natural

For our mind.

2. Healing in Naturopathy and Ayurveda:-Both systems appreciate the natural tendency of our body to heal. Outer remedies and procedures help to support our inner Core to recover and it's ability to heal the body and condition. Naturopathy emphasizes the vital force and it's ability to heal the body and mind. Ayurveda further assists the inner vital force by actively resorting the imbalances in our tissues and humours and by actively detoxifying the body.

3.Mind and psychological health in Naturopathy and Ayurveda:--The concept of mind and consciousness and it's integration with body is one of the fundamental feature of Naturopathy as well as Ayurveda. As we have Ayurveda body types based on 3 humor or doshas, there are different mind types in Ayurveda based on 3 primary psychological attributes. Satva, Rajas, Tamas.

4.Concept of detox in Naturopathy and Ayurveda:-our body is constantly detoxified everyday through sweating, breathing, passing urine and stool, and sometimes vomiting and at the level of whole body. Naturopathy assists this process of natural detoxification via it's different modalities of treatment as fasting, diet or organic food, sweating, cold and hot treatments, mud therapy, sun bath and massage for correcting the imbalance of humors and restoration of health. The Ayurvedic panchkarma therapy goes one step ahead and deals with the impacted humors in the deeper levels of various tissues. It is facilitated or Induced Detoxification of Ayurvedic Medicine.

5.Preventive and health promoting measures in Naturopathy and Ayurveda:-Ayurveda as well as Naturopathy can be used even when the person is healthy or to prevent any particular disorder to which a person is susceptible. In Ayurvedic medicine, some rejuvenative remedies are described that are used to promote overall health or the health of a particular organ or to correct a particular condition are known by the name "Rasayan".

Natural Diet :- Food is considered as medicine in naturopathy. The natural food helps to eliminate the toxins deposited in the body and enhance the vital energy immunity.

Types of food or diet:-In naturopathy there are 2 types of food I. e, positive and negative.

Positive (primary food) :-1.Healthy food

2.Alkaline in nature

3.Light and easily digestible

4.Rich in cellulose or roughage

5.Rich in vitamin and minerals

6.Helps to elimination the toxins from the body

7.Non mucus food

8.examples:-vegetables, fruits

Negative (secondary food) :-1.Unhealthy food

2.Acidic in nature

3.Heavy and constipating

4.Refined food.

5.Rich in carbohydrates, protein and fat

6.promotes accumulation of the toxins in the body

7.Mucus producing food

8.examples:-cereals, pulses, milk, egg, nuts, non vegetarian food.

Health promoting rules of diet in naturopathy:-

1.Diet should be taken at fixed timings usually twice a day

2.Diet should not be taken unless the previous diet is already digested

3.Nothing should be taken between the meals, frequent eating and overeating causes indigestion.

4.Adequatly chewing of food is necessary, it makes the food digestible.

5.During the meal one should be happy and quiet.

6.water should be taken in less quantity with meal.

7.Fruits and salad should be compulsory ingredient of diet.

Pandemic or epidemic:-pandemic is described in charak viman sthan chapter 3.it is

*Mentioned that when any disease contaminate
air ,country,season,water of any special place and spread very rapidly is called pandemic or epidemic*

In charaksamitha it is mentioned about symptoms of contaminated air:- this air is very unhealthy it flows against the season it means it will flows in a very rapid way or either very slow way or very dry,very cold,very hot,very moist,it comes from different directions and met with each other, full of dust

Symptoms of contaminated water:- it has foul smell, colour and touch is moist. The birds who live in water leave the ponds or that area and the ponds,seas where the birds animals live they leave that area and they even died there the taste of that water is not tasty

As we all know that this pandemic covid-19 corona virus changed our life we become more aware about our health. But how many of us know that it had been already mentioned in our anctient books by sushrut samihita(father of surgery). In india it is mentioned earlier about the pandemic and about their courses and symptoms and treatment also. According to sushrut samihita in 5th chapter 33-38 shloka it is mentioned about how this

Goals of life

1.Many problems will come into our life but we will not complain because god is a type of a director who gave very tough role to his best actor

2. Everything is possible in this world and every person has that quality, energy and power to make every impossible thing to make possible everyone can stand in first row and can write history from his work and energy.

3. It is the cheerful mind that is preserving it is the strong mind that hews its way through a thousand difficulties.

4.Life is priceless to live life for small goals is the shame for life

5. Till there is life in human body person should not be sad or leaving hope because continuously if we try to reach the goal one day we will definitely get success.

6.never lose faith in yourself you can do anything in the universe

7. those who live for others really live and those who live only for themselves are more dead than alive

8. Oh, to live even for a day in the full light of freedom to breath the free air of simplicity isn't that the highest purity?

9.if you think that you are bound. You remain bound. you make your own bondage. If you know that you are free. You are free this moment this is knowledge of freedom freedom is the goal of all nature.

10. Freedom can never be reached by the weak. Throw away all weakness. Tell your body that it is strong. Tell your mind that it is strong. and have unbound faith and hope in yourself.

11. All the knowledge that the world has ever received comes from the mind. The infinite library of the universe is in our own mind.

12. stand up be bold be strong. Take the whole responsibility on your own shoulder and know that you are the creator of your own destiny. All the strength and success you want is within yourselves therefore make your own future.

13.if you want to be a yogi you must be free and place yourself in circumstances where you are alone and free from all anxiety. The one who desires a comfortable and nice life and at the same time wants to realize the atman is like the fool who wanting to cross the river caught hold of a crocodile mistaking it for a log of a wood.

14. in the world take always the position of the giver give everything and look for no return. Give love, give help, give service, give any little thing you can but keep our barter. Make no conditions and non will be imposed. Let us give our own bounty. Just as god gives to us.

15. give up all desires for enjoyment in earth or heaven. Control the organs of the senses and control the mind. Bear every misery without even knowing that you are miserable. Think of nothing but spiritual freedom.

16. the whole secret of existance is to have no fear. Never fear what will become of you depend on no one only the moment you regect all help are you free.

17. tell the truth boldly whether It hurts or not. Never pander to weakness. If truth is too much for people and sweeps them away let them go the sooner the better.

18. take up one idea. Make that one idea your life. Think of it. Dream of it. Live on that idea. Let the brain, muscles, nerves every part of your body be full of that idea and just leave every other idea alone .This is the way to success that is the way great spiritual giants are produced.

19.Each work has to pass through these stages ridicule opposition and then acceptance.Those who think a head of their time are sure to be misunderstood.

20. In a day when you donot come across any problems you can be sure that you are travelling on the wrong path.

21.Anything that brings spiritual,mental or physical weakness touch it not with the toes of your feet.

22.To succeed you must have tremendous preservance tremendous will "I will drink the ocean at my will mountains will crumble up" says .the preserving soul have that sort of energy that sort of will work hard and you will reach the goal.

23.All power is within You.You can do anything and everything .Believe in that Do not believe that you are weak do not belive that you are half crazy lunatics as most of us do nowdays.

24.Do not look back upon what has been done Go ahead!

25. by doing well the duty which is nearest to us the duty which is in our hands now we make ourselves stronger and improving our strength in this manner step by step we may reach a state in which it shall be our privilege to do the most coveted and honoured duties in life and in society.

26. let us make our hearts as big as the ocean to go beyond all the trifles of the world and see it only as a picture we can then enjoy the world without being in anyway affected by it.

27. superstition is our great every bigotry is worse.

28. if you want to have life you have to die every moment for it. Life and death are only different expressions of the same thing looked at from different standpoints they are the falling and the rising of the same wave and the 2 form one whole

29. is there any sex-distinction in the 'Atman' or self? Out with the differentiation between man and women all is 'atman'! give up the identification with the body and standup!

30. in judging others we always judge them by our own ideals that is not as it should be

YOGA AND LIFESTYLE:- Indeed,it is an astonishing fact that a yogic tradition ,which is more than 5 thousand years old,has recently become a popular way of life .Presently,people consider that yoga is a significant means to achieve a healthy as well as a positive lifestyle.In fact ,the power of yoga lies in its simplicity,flexibility and diversity.As a matter of fact ,yoga helps in improving our flexibility, lowers our stress level and increases our confidence and finally contributes to a healthier lifestyle on the whole.There are various lifestyle diseases like obesity,diabetes,asthma,HTN,back pain,migraine and depression which can be prevented and treated up to some extent with the help of certain yogic exercise.

ASANAS AS preventive MEASURES:- Asan means "sthiram sukham asanam" i.e,"that position which is comfortable and steady." In Brahaman upanishad, "To sit in a comfortable position or posture for everlasting period is called ASANA.ASANA is that state of body in which the body may be positioned easily .As a matter of fact ,the ability to be sit comfortably for an extended period of time in any position is called ASANA.

In ASANAS ,body is kept in various positions in such a way that the activities of organs and glands of body become more efficient and eventually the health of mind and body is improved.

Infact ,Asan is a means through which physical and mental development is achieved .prevention of diseases and delay in ageing and mental development is achieved .Prevention of diseases and delay in ageing are the desired effects that can be achieved through yogic exercises.There are different types of Asanas which include meditative asanas ,relaxative asanas and corrective asanas.Regular practice of the above -mentioned asanas significantly affects various systems or organs of our body .Asanas can be used as preventive measures because they provide the following physiological benefits ,which ultimately help us in avoiding various life style diseases such as diabetes ,obesity and cardio-vascular diseases.

Benefits of Asanas for prevention of Diseases:-a.Bones and joints Become strong:-As a result of performing asanas regularly ,the bones ,cartilages and ligaments become strong .

Along with this ,the height of children is enhanced .The joints are able to bear more pressure.Asanas also enhance the flexibility of joints.

The flexibility of spine is also enhanced .Postural deformities can also be prevented and corrected.

Arthritis is also cured by performing asanas .Due to spinal injuries problems like back pain ,sciatica and cervical pain develop .By performing asanas these problems are greatly controlled.

b.Muscles Become strong:-By performing asanas regularly,muscles of the body become strong .The efficiency of muscles increases.Fat doesnot accumulate in the body.

49

c. Circulation of Blood Becomes Normal:-As a result of practicing asanas regularly,the stroke volume as well as cardiac output increase because cardiac muscles start working more strongly and efficiently .Blood circulation is improved and blood pressure normalises and stabilises.The level of blood cholestrol reduces .By performing asanas ,the lactic acid and acid phosphate are excreted from muscles quickly and easily which reduces fatigue.

d.Respiratory Organs Become Efficient :-By doing asanas regularly ,the respiratory organs become efficient .The vital air capacity increases up to 6000 cc..The size of the lungs and chest also enhances .As a result of doing asanas ,the will power becomes strong and various disease such as cough ,asthma and cancer of trachea can be prevented.

e.Efficiency of Digestive System Increases :- By performing asanas regularly all the organs of digestive system of our body begin to work effectively .The absorption of food becomes efficient.The storage of bile in gall bladder in concentrated form is enhanced appetite increases ,stomach and intestines are also strengthened .,constipation,indigestion and gas trouble are reduced.

f.Nervous System Strengthens:- As a result of regular practice of asanas ,our nervous system strengthens .The working efficiency of synapse enhances.The neuro -muscular coordination increases.

Activities of our body will be done expending less energy .The secretion adrenaline depends on sympathetic nervous system .The reaction time also reduces .Mental power also improves .Memory improvez and feeling of dissapointment

OBESITY:- Now days ,obesity has become an enormous as well as fatal hralth problem .This problem is not only seen in India but is prevalent in the other countries is also .Even in the United states of America ,one out of three adults and one out of 5 children and teenagers are facing the problem of obesity.In India,we witness a similar situation.Majority of the people,since childhood,fall prey to obesity is most of the countries of the world ."Obesity is that condition of the body in which the amount of fat increases to extreme levels.In others words,obrsity can be defined as "the condition when an individualvweighs 20% more than the ideal weight."An adult with a BMI more than or equal to 30 than the ideal BMI is usually considered to be obese. In case of obesity, the body weight of the individual is always more in comparison to height. Considering the number of health risks associated with obesity ,it has been declared a diseases.It has been observed that obese persons usually fall prey to diabetes,hypertension,cardiovascular diseases ,cancer,arthrities,osteoarthritis,flat foot,resperatory problems,varicose veins,liver malfunction etc.Generally,the questions arise:-What should be the ideal body weight of an individual?Who is obese and who is not?Different methods are used in different countries to know if an individual is obese.According to the first method ,just by observing ,it can be inferred whether he or she is obse ot not.But this method cannot be considered a right method to determine if an individual is obese because the opinion about the shape of the body changes with the passage of time.for example,chubbiness used to be liked bg people in yesteryears,whereas being slim and trim is appreciated nowdays everywhere .According to the second method ,if an individual's body weight is more in proportion to his/her height ,the individual will be overweight or obese.But this method cannot be accepted as the best method .The 3rd method is a morevscientific method .In this method ,the body fat percentage is calculated .If the body fat percentage of a person is more than the required levels, he /she may be considered obese .This is the most accurate methid tovdtermine obesity,but it is not easy to apply this method.In comparision to other methods ,the weight and height chart is still preferred to determine obesiry because it is easily available,cost-effective and easy to use.Another method to check obesity is using BMI(Body Mass Index).If you want to know your body mass index,then divide your body weight in kg by your height in meter square viz.

Body Mass Index=weight in kg÷height inmetere square=weight in kg ÷height ×height

Obesity can be prevented as well as cured if the following asanas are performed regularly

1.Vajrasan

Procedure:-It is a meditative asana.Kneel down on the ground floor with your knees,ankles and toes touching the ground .Your toes should be stretched backwards.Now place your palms of your hands on the knees.The upper body should be straight.At this time,the breathing should be deep,even and slow.Then expand your chest forward and pull your abdominal portion inwards.

Benefits:-1.It is helpful in improving concentration

2.It is helpful in curing dysentry ,back pain and chest disease.

3.It enhances memory power.

4.It cures the problems related to menstruation.

5.It cures mental stress.

6.It strengthens the pelvic muscles.

7.It removes postural defect.

8.It prevents hernia and gives relief from piles.

9.It is the best asana for people suffering from sciatica and sacral infections.

10.It helps in reducing hi fat.

2.PADAHASTASANA

Procedure:-Bend forward until the fingers or palms of the hands touch the floor on either side of the feet .Try to touch the knees with the forehead.

Do not strain .keep the knees straight.Exhale while bending forward .Try to contract the abdomen in the final position to expek,the maximum amount of air from the lungs.

BENEFITS

1.Patahastasana makes the body very flexible.It stretches the back and leg muscles.

2.It helps to determinate excess belly fat.

3.It improves digestion and reduces constipation .It cures many stomach ailments.

4.It makes the spine flexible anf tones the nerves

5.It improves blood circulation

CONTRA-INDICATION

1.The individuals who have back pain should avoid this asana.At least,they shouldnot bend fotward fully.They can bend themselves only as far as vomfortable.

3.URDHVA HASTASANA

Procedure:- You must begin by assuming Tadasana.Stand with your arms at your sides.Then ,gently raise them to the ceiling .Make sure that your arms are parallel to each other.You can also bring your palms together over your head.While you do this ,make sure your shoulders are not touched.

If your palms are a part,then they must face each other.Your arms must be straight at all times such that they are activated all throughout,must be away from your ears and your shoulders blades must be pressed firmly on your back .Your thighs should be engaged in such a way that they pull the kneecaps up.Straighten your legs,but do not lock your knees.

BENEFITS

4.Trikonasana

Procedure:- First of all stand with your legs apart.Then raise the arms sideways up to the shoulder level.Bend the trunk sideways and raise the right hand upward .Touch the ground with left hand behind left foot.After sometime ,do the same asana with opposite arm in the same way.

BENEFITS

1.It strengthens the legs,knees,armd and chest

2.It helps in improving digestion and stimulatez all the abdominal organs.

3.It increases mental and physical equilibrium

Gomukhasana:-

Procedure:- sit down on the ground with legs stretched forward .Now fold the left leg at knee and sit on the left foot .Fold the right leg and keep the right thigh on the left thigh with the help of your hands.Now lift your buttocks and bring the heels of both feet togethet so that they should touch each other.Now fold your left arm behind your back over the shoulder.Fold the right arm behind the back under the right shouldet.After that bend your fingets of both the hands and clasp each other.At this time your head and back should be erect.Then repeat the same in reverse position.

Benefits:-1.It makes the leg muscles strong and elastic

2.It improves the function of lungs

3.It also reduces stress and anxiety

4.It improves the function of kidneys by stimulating it thushelps the individuals who suffer from diabetes

Contraindication:-1.The individual who suffer from shoulder,knee or back pain should avoid this asana

2.Avoid this asan in case of any knee injury

3.Avoid this asan in case of recent or chronic knee or hip injury or inflammation

Bhujangasan

Procedure:- In this asana,the shape of the body remains like snake that's is why it is called bhujangasan .In order to perform this asama lie down on the belly on the ground.keep your hands near the shoulders.keep your hands near the shoulders .keep your legs close together.Now straighten up yout arms slowly ,raise the chrst .Your head should be backwards.Keep this position for some time.Then come to former position.For good results,perform this asana 3-5 times

Benefits:-1.It alleviates obesity

2.It provides strength and agility

3.It cures the disease of liver

4.It improves blood circulation

5.It makes the vertebral column flexible and thin

Contraindication:-1.This asana should be avoided by people who suffer from hernia ,back injuries,headache,and recent abdominal surgeries

2.Pregnant women should not perform this asana.

Vakrasan

Procedure:-sit down and stretch your legs straight.Fold the right leg and keep the right leg's heel touching the leg's knee.Place your right hand behind your back and left arm over the right knee;hold your right ankle.Push your right knee as far as possible anf while exhaling ,twist yout trunk to the right side.Take sufficient support of left arm.Now,repeat the same procedure with the left side.

Benefits:-1.It prevents and control diabetes.

2.It improves the function of both spinal cord and nervous system

3.It reduces belly fat

4.It strengthens kidneys.

5.It gives relief in stiffness of vertebrae.

Contraindication:-1.Avoid this asana in case of high blood pressure

2.Individuals who suffer from peptic ulcer should not do this asana

3.This asana should not be performed who suffer from serious back injury.

STRESS:- life would be simple indeed if our needs could always be satisfied.Stress is not new to human beings .It has existed throughout human evolution.At work or in day to day life,everyone experiences stress.Millions of trials and errors in the life process have brought human beings to this stage.We know that there are many obstacles in our life which interfere with gratification of our needs and complicate our efforts towards our goals.we all face delays,deprivation,failures,losses,restrictions,obligation,illness,conflicts,pressure etc.such events place stress on us which may be very harmful to us .so it becomes important for us to know the exact meaning of stress.

Meaning of stress:- stress consists of bodily changes produced by physiological or psycological conditions that tend to upset the homostatic balance.In medical language stress is defined as perturfation of the body's homostatis.

Types of stress:-Most of thestress situation we face in everyday life are very minor and easy to cope with.example where we feel hungry we may stop what we are doing and go to take a meal .we can meet such demands very easily .That is why we are not disturbed physiologicaly.Generally such type of stress is caused by physical stressors such as diet ,exercise,illness,noise,extremes of temperature etc.

Stress management techniques:-There are no. of stress management techniques such as change in lifestyle,relaxation techniqurs like meditation,yogic exercise,physical exercises,listening to soothing music,deep breathing,massage etc.These techniques have positive effect on reducing stress.some techniques which are easy to use ate mentioned below:-1.Participation in physical Activities:-When you face stressful situation you should engage yourself in regular physical activity or exercise.This can manage the stress effectively and efficiently .The exercise should be of moderate to high intensity.Aerobic exercises are good for reducing stress.Physical activitu is one of the best means of releasing stress.

It increases the fitness of individuals .Indeed it has been observed that the individual who are physically fit have a better health status.Such people are more resistany the effects of stress than less physically fit person.

2.Achieve a high level of physical fitness:- for proper management of stress it is important to achieve high level of physical fitness .The goal of stress management is to use stress advantageously not to eliminate all stress from one's life .Too little or too severe stress tend to lower our performance.

3.Cognitive stratigies to change the perception of the stressor:-The individual who is unfer stress should use cognitive strategies to change the perception of the stressor.He should analyse the situation of stress.He should consider the stressor as a challenge rather than a threat .He should have positive thinking towards the stress.

4.Building self confidence:- An individual under stress should try to build his/her selfconfidence.He /she should have enough confidence to deal with stress.

5.Relaxation Techniques:-Are very effective in reducing stress for physical relaxation,one should undertake various physical education programmes.Ifa person perform some exercises for legs ,his muscles of legs wil be tense after that other muscle group should be exercised so that the muscles of legs could be relaxed.

6.Developing Hobbies:- Developing various type of hobbies ,such as gardening,tv
watching ,swimming,listening to music is also significant for reducing stress.

7.staying cool and confident under pressure:-One should try to stay cool and confident when there is stress.Remaining in such a state can be helpful in reducing stress.

8.Avoid the company of stressed persons:- Stressed people usually remain busy in talking about thrir own stress. They become pessimistic .You can be affected by their veiws .So always avoid such people who remain under stress.

9.Don't Think about stressful thoughts:-It has been observed that most of the people always remain worried for no reason.In fact ,most of these things might never happen in life .so ,why waste all our energy worrying needlessly.

In conclusion ,it can be said that stress can be reduced or managed properly with the help of the above-mentioned points.